Human Anatomy
COLORING BOOK

The Complete Anatomy & Physiology Coloring Workbook
For Adults, Nurses, and Medical Students

WITH COMPLETE SOLUTIONS

THIS BOOK
BELONGS TO:

_____

_____

_____

_____

The Skull - (Anterior View)

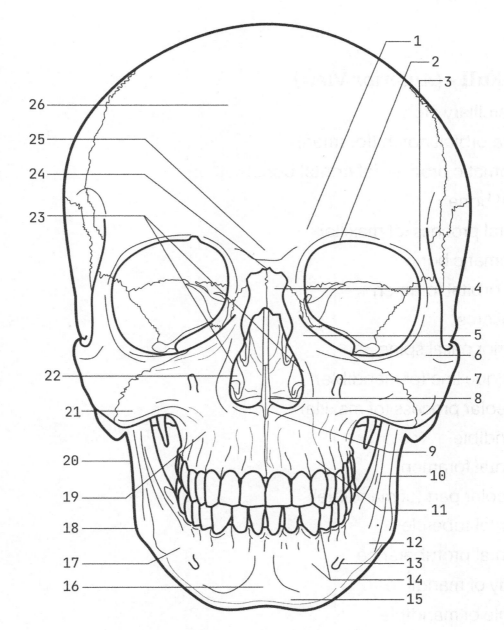

1 _____
2 _____
3 _____
4 _____
5 _____
6 _____
7 _____
8 _____
9 _____
10 _____
11 _____
12 _____
13 _____

14 _____
15 _____
16 _____
17 _____
18 _____
19 _____
20 _____
21 _____
22 _____
23 _____
24 _____
25 _____
26 _____

The Skull - *(Anterior View)*

1. Superciliary arch
2. Supra-orbital notch (foramen)
3. Zygomatic process (of frontal bone)
4. Nasal bone
5. Frontal process (of maxilla)
6. Zygomatic bone
7. Infra-orbital foramen
8. Nasal crest
9. Anterior nasal spine
10. Oblique line (of mandible)
11. Alveolar process (of maxilla)
12. Mandible
13. Mental foramen
14. Alveolar part (of mandible)
15. Mental tubercle
16. Mental protuberance
17. Body of mandible
18. Angle of mandible
19. Maxilla
20. Ramus of mandible
21. Zygomatic process (of maxilla)
22. Inferior nasal concha
23. Piriform aperture
24. Nasion
25. Glabella
26. Frontal bone

The Skull - *(Lateral View)*

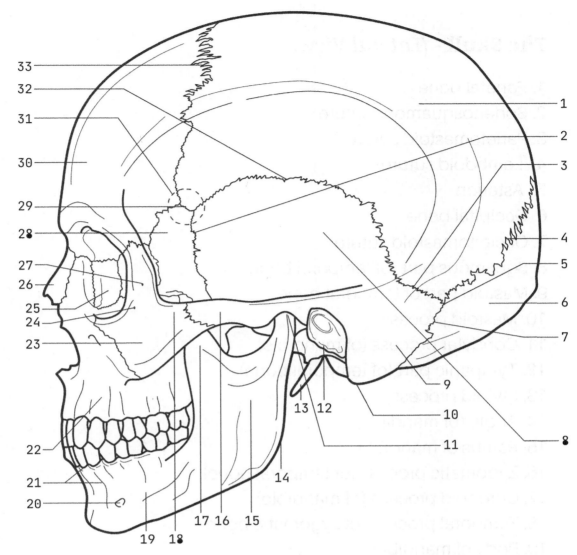

1 _____	18 _____
2 _____	19 _____
3 _____	20 _____
4 _____	21 _____
5 _____	22 _____
6 _____	23 _____
7 _____	24 _____
8 _____	25 _____
9 _____	26 _____
10 _____	27 _____
11 _____	28 _____
12 _____	29 _____
13 _____	30 _____
14 _____	31 _____
15 _____	32 _____
16 _____	33 _____
17 _____	

The Skull - *(Lateral View)*

1. Parietal bone
2. Sphenosquamous suture
3. Parietomastoid suture
4. Lambdoid suture
5. Asterion
6. Occipital bone
7. Occipitomastoid suture
8. Squamous part (of temporal bone)
9. Mastoid part of temporal bone
10. Mastoid process
11. Condylar process (of mandible)
12. Tympanic part (of temporal bone)
13. Styloid process
14. Angle (of mandible)
15. Ramus of mandible
16. Zygomatic process (of temporal bone)
17. Coronoid process (of mandible)
18. Temporal process (of zygomatic bone)
19. Body of mandible
20. Mental foramen
21. Alveolar part (of mandible)
22. Maxilla
23. Zygomatic bone
24. Zygomaticofacial foramen
25. Lacrimal bone
26. Nasal bone
27. Zygomaticotemporal foramen (on deep surface of zygomatic bone)
28. Greater wing (of sphenoid bone)
29. Sphenoparietal suture
30. Frontal bone
31. Pterion
32. Squamous suture
33. Coronal suture

The Skull - (Posterior View)

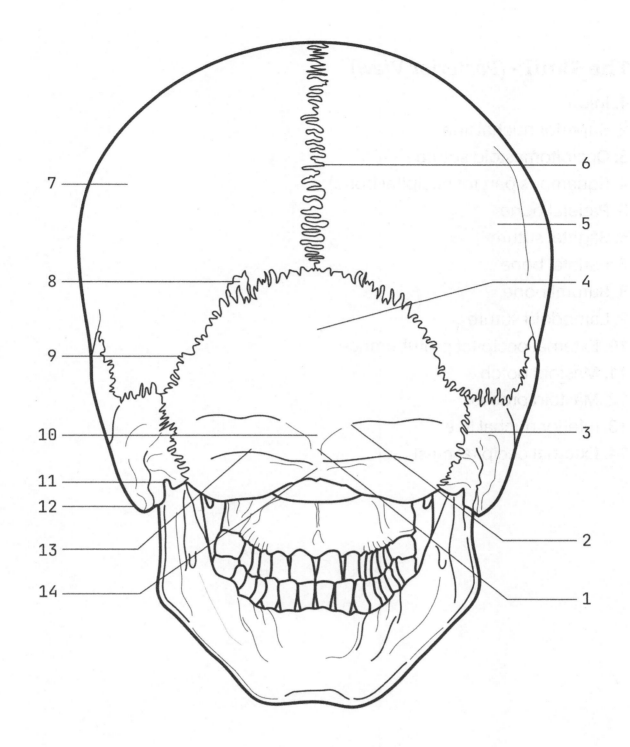

1 _____ 8 _____

2 _____ 9 _____

3 _____ 10 _____

4 _____ 11 _____

5 _____ 12 _____

6 _____ 13 _____

7 _____ 14 _____

The Skull - *(Posterior View)*

1. Inion
2. Superior nuchal line
3. Occipitomastoid suture
4. Squamous part (of occipital bone)
5. Parietal bone
6. Sagittal suture
7. Parietal bone
8. Sutural bone
9. Lambdoid suture
10. External occipital protuberance
11. Mastoid notch
12. Mastoid process
13. Inferior nuchal line
14. External occipital crest

The Skull - (Superior View)

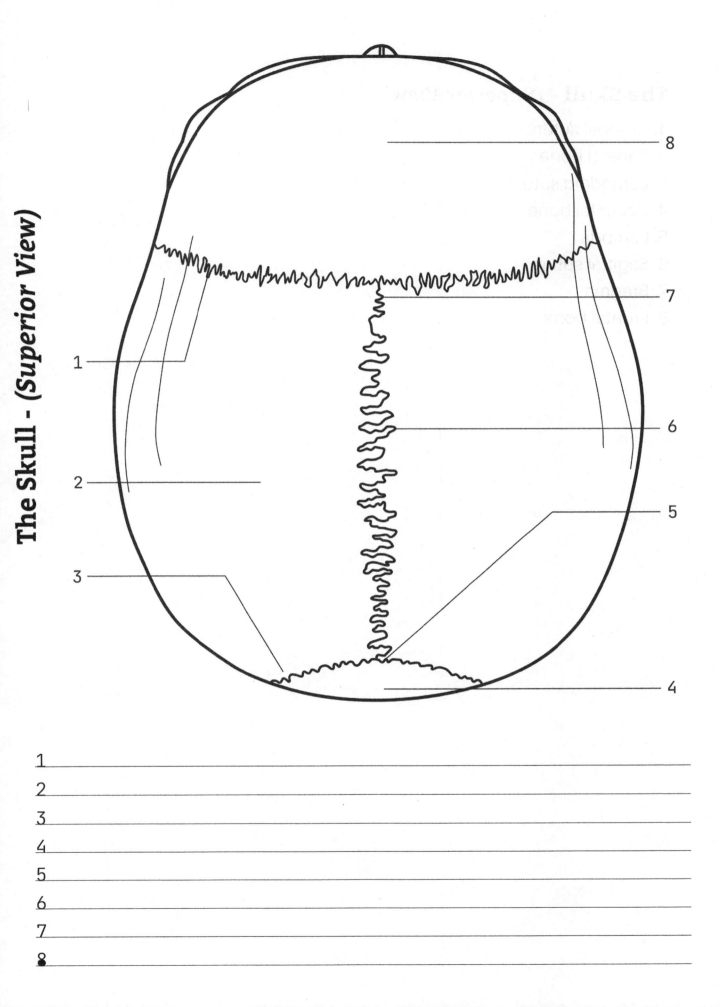

1 _____

2 _____

3 _____

4 _____

5 _____

6 _____

7 _____

8 _____

The Skull - *(Superior View)*

1. Coronal suture
2. Parietal bone
3. Lambdoid suture
4. Occipital bone
5. Lambda
6. Sagittal suture
7. Bregma
8. Frontal bone

Facial Muscles - (Lateral View)

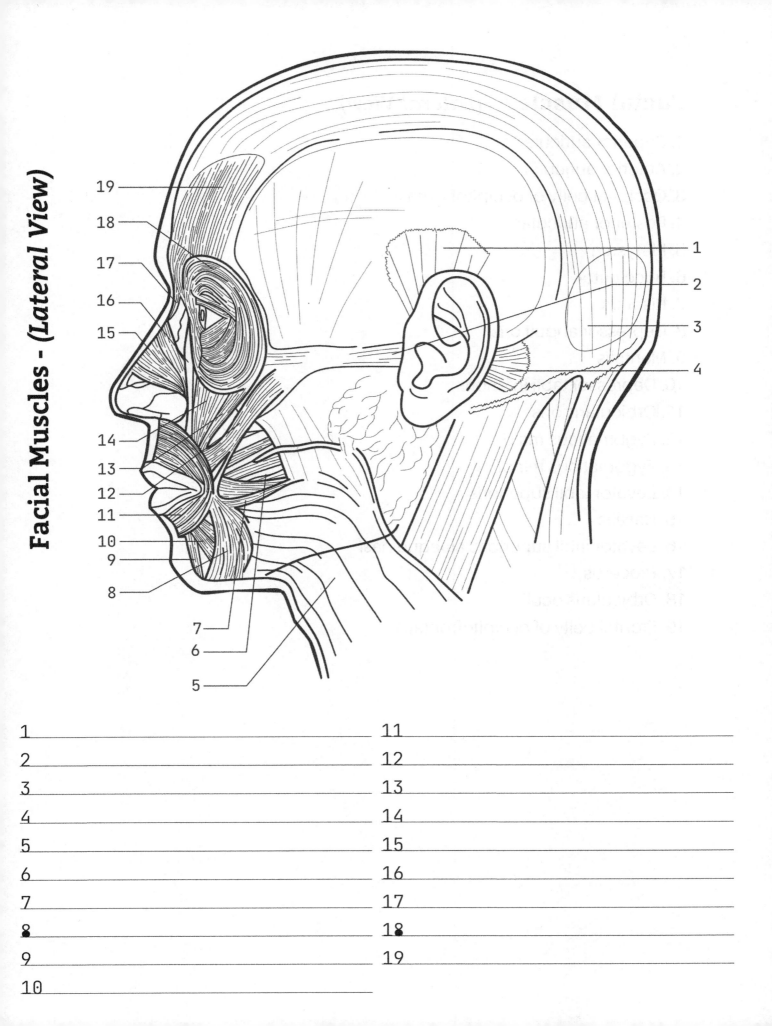

1 _____   11 _____
2 _____   12 _____
3 _____   13 _____
4 _____   14 _____
5 _____   15 _____
6 _____   16 _____
7 _____   17 _____
8 _____   18 _____
9 _____   19 _____
10 _____

Facial Muscles - *(Lateral View)*

1. Superior auricular
2. Anterior auricular
3. Occipital belly of occipitofrontalis
4. Posterior auricular
5. Platysma
6. Buccinator
7. Risorius
8. Depressor anguli oris
9. Mentalis
10. Depressor labii inferioris
11. Orbicularis oris
12. Zygomaticus major
13. Zygomaticus minor
14. Levator labii superioris
15. Nasalis
16. Levator labii superioris alaeque nasi
17. Procerus
18. Orbicularis oculi
19. Frontal belly of occipitofrontalis

External Ear

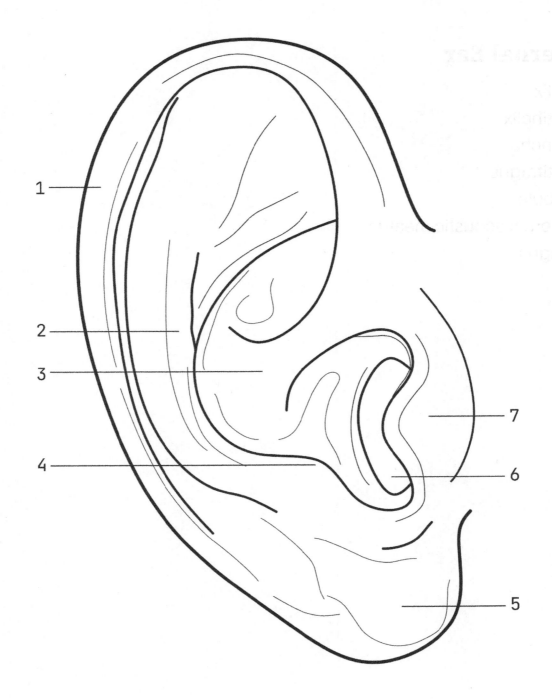

1 _____

2 _____

3 _____

4 _____

5 _____

6 _____

7 _____

External Ear

1. Helix
2. Antihelix
3. Concha
4. Antitragus
5. Lobule
6. External acoustic meatus
7. Tragus

External, Middle, and Inner Ear

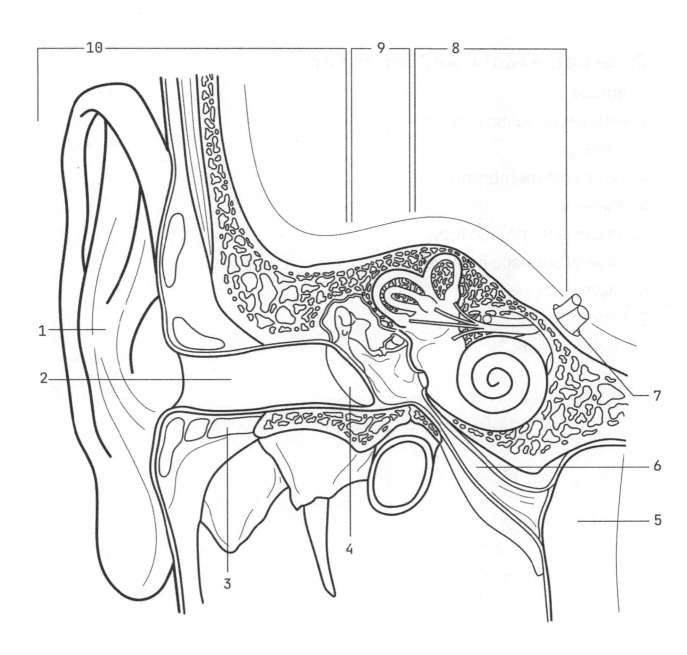

1 _____

2 _____

3 _____

4 _____

5 _____

6 _____

7 _____

8 _____

9 _____

10 _____

External, Middle, and Inner Ear

1. Auricle
2. External acoustic meatus
3. Cartilage
4. Tympanic membrane
5. Pharynx
6. Pharyngotympanic tube
7. Internal acoustic meatus
8. Internal ear
9. Middle ear
10. External ear

The Structure of the Internal Ear

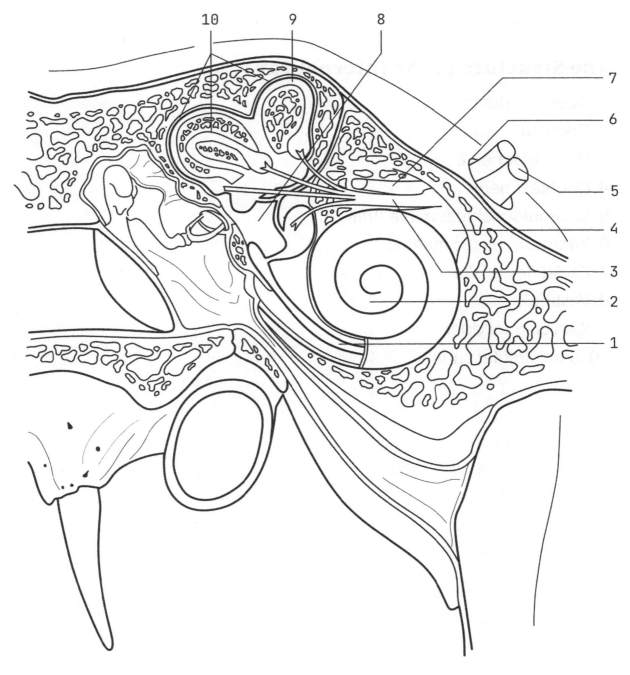

1 _____

2 _____

3 _____

4 _____

5 _____

6 _____

7 _____

8 _____

9 _____

10 _____

The Structure of the Internal Ear

1. Cochlear duct
2. Cochlea
3. Vestibular nerve
4. Cochlear nerve
5. Vestibulocochlear nerve [VIII]
6. Internal acoustic meatus
7. Facial nerve [VII]
8. Vestibule
9. Semicircular duct
10. Semicircular canals

Overview of Oral Cavity

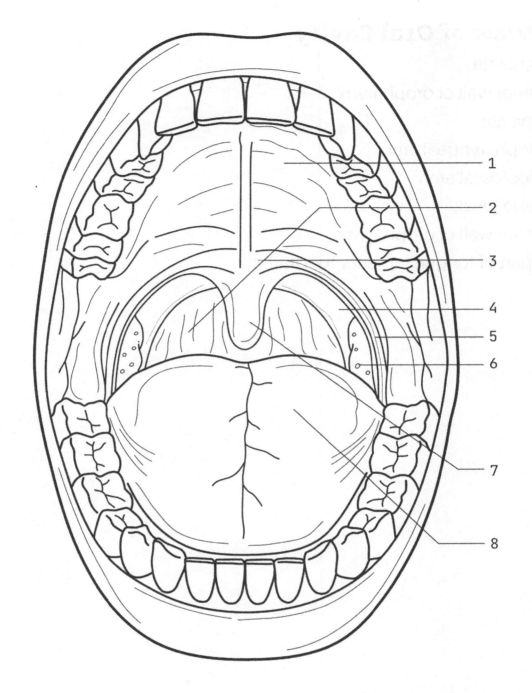

1   _____
2   _____
3   _____
4   _____
5   _____
6   _____
7   _____

1   _____
2   _____
3   _____
4   _____
5   _____
6   _____
7   _____
8   _____

Overview of Oral Cavity

1. Hard palate
2. Posterior wall of oropharynx
3. Soft palate
4. Palatopharyngeal arch
5. Palatoglossal arch
6. Palatine tonsil
7. Posterior wall of oropharynx
8. Oral part of tongue (anterior two thirds)

Thoracic Skeleton

1 _____

2 _____

3 _____

Thoracic Skeleton

1. True ribs I to VII
2. False ribs VIII to XII
3. Floating ribs XI and XII

Mediastinum - Subdivisions

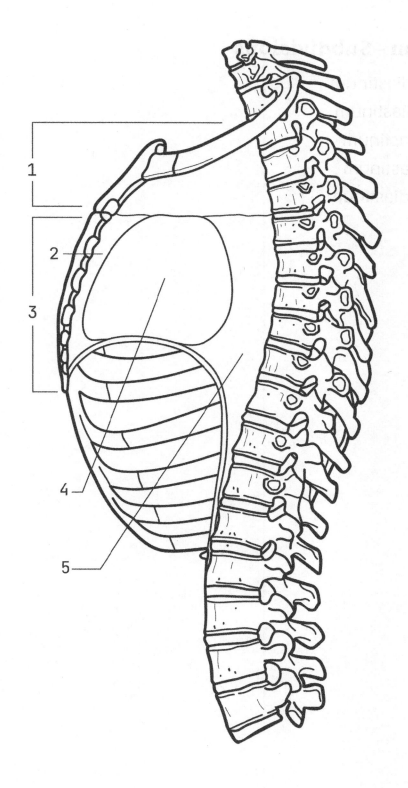

1 _____

2 _____

3 _____

4 _____

5 _____

Mediastinum - Subdivisions

1. Superior mediastinum
2. Anterior mediastinum
3. Inferior mediastinum
4. Middle mediastinum
5. Posterior mediastinum

Pericardium

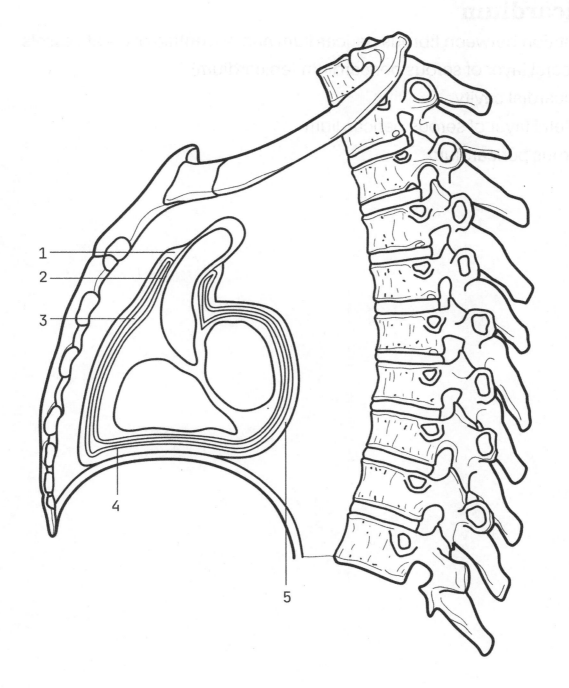

1 _____

2 _____

3 _____

4 _____

5 _____

Pericardium

1. Junction between fibrous pericardium and adventitia of great vessels
2. Visceral layer of serous pericardium (epicardium)
3. Pericardial cavity
4. Parietal layer of serous pericardium
5. Fibrous pericardium

Vertebra, Ribs and Sternum

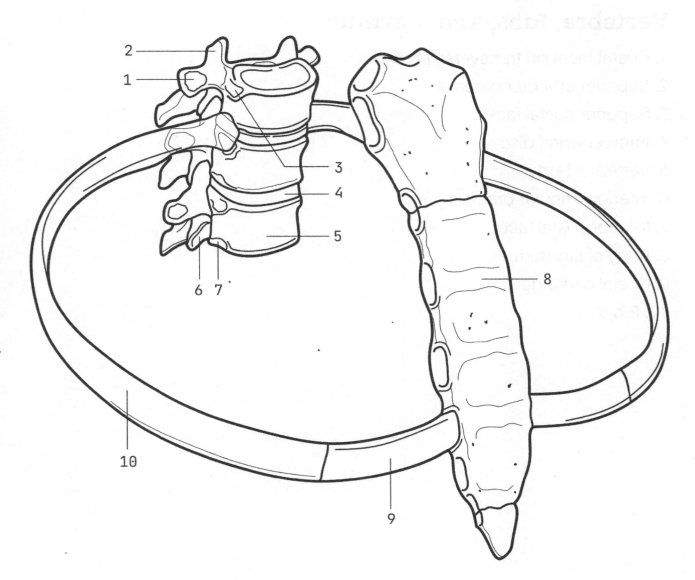

1 _____

2 _____

3 _____

4 _____

5 _____

6 _____

7 _____

8 _____

9 _____

10 _____

Vertebra, Ribs, and Sternum

1. Costal facet on transverse process
2. Superior articular process
3. Superior costal facet
4. Intervertebral disc
5. Vertebral body
6. Inferior articular process
7. Inferior costal facet
8. Body of sternum
9. Costal cartilage
10. Rib V

Sternum

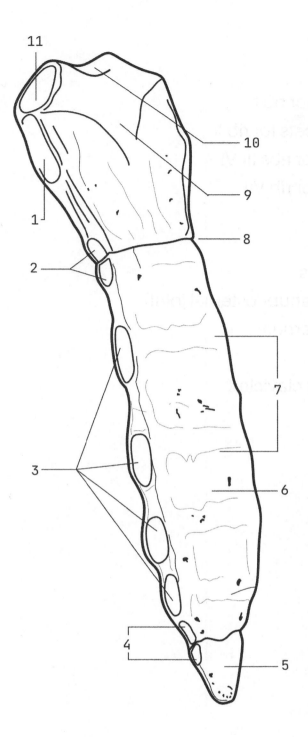

1 _____   7 _____

2 _____   8 _____

3 _____   9 _____

4 _____   10 _____

5 _____   11 _____

6 _____

Sternum

1. Attachment site for rib I
2. Articular demifacets for rib II
3. Articular facets for ribs III-VI
4. Articular facets for rib VII
5. Xiphoid process
6. Body of sternum
7. Transverse ridges
8. Sternal angle (manubriosternal joint)
9. Manubrium of sternum
10. Jugular notch
11. Articular site for clavicle

Typical Rib

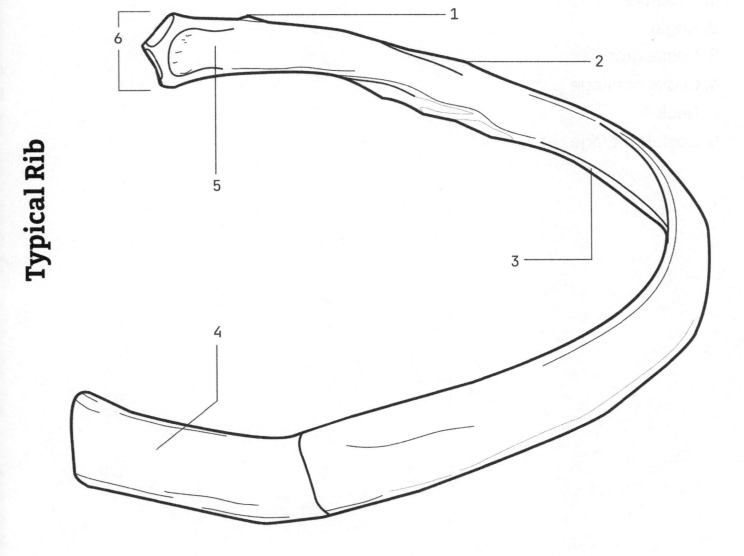

1 _____

2 _____

3 _____

4 _____

5 _____

6 _____

Typical Rib

1. Tubercle
2. Angle
3. Costal groove
4. Costal cartilage
5. Neck
6. Costal cartilage

Thoracic Cavity

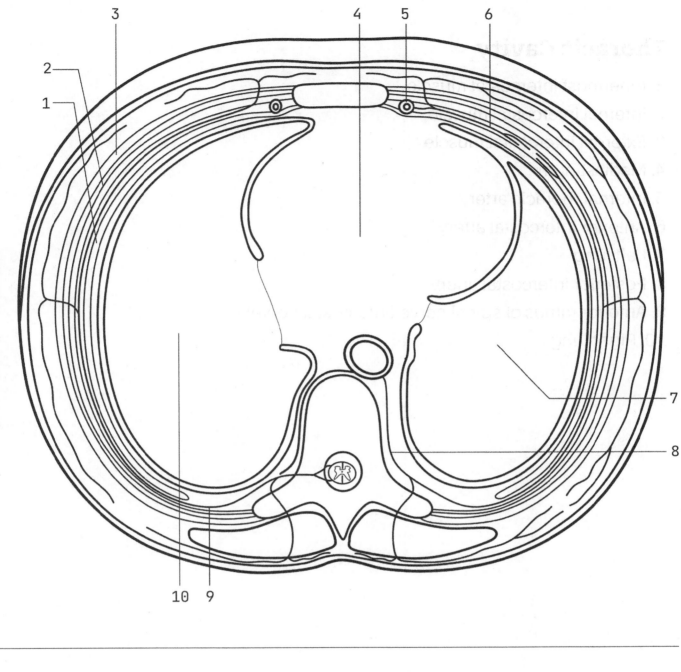

1 _____

2 _____

3 _____

4 _____

5 _____

6 _____

7 _____

8 _____

9 _____

10 _____

Thoracic Cavity

1. Innermost intercostal muscle
2. Internal intercostal muscle
3. External intercostal muscle
4. Mediastinum
5. Internal thoracic artery
6. Anterior intercostal artery
7. Left lung
8. Posterior intercostal artery
9. Anterior ramus of spinal nerve (intercostal nerve)
10. Right lung

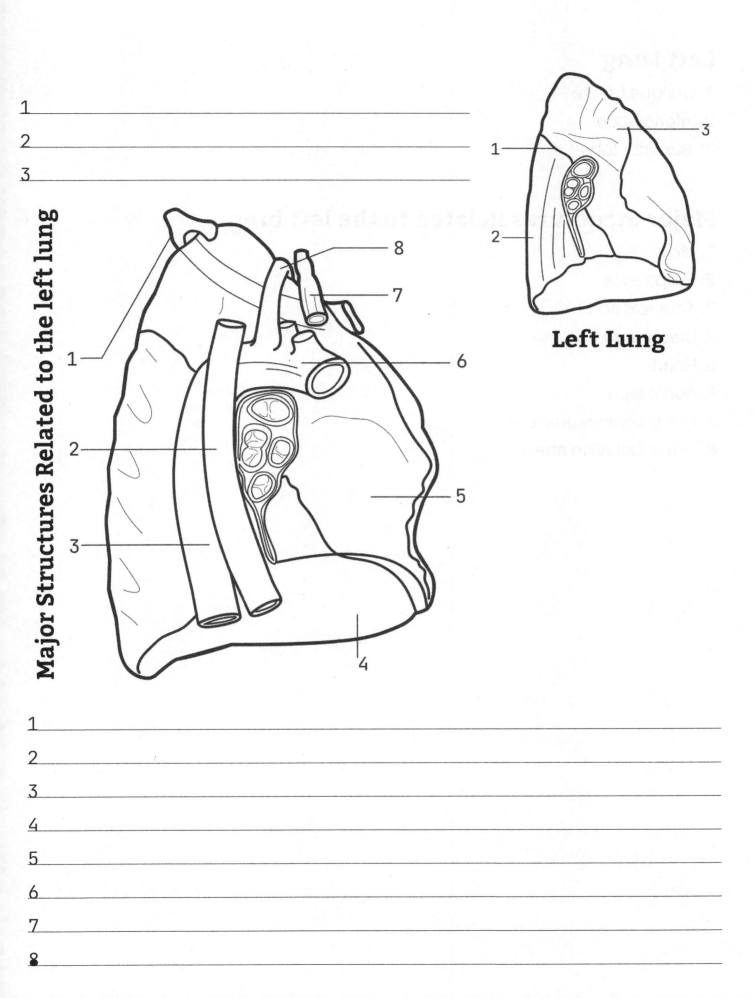

1 _____

2 _____

3 _____

Left Lung

Major Structures Related to the left lung

1 _____

2 _____

3 _____

4 _____

5 _____

6 _____

7 _____

8 _____

Left Lung

1. Oblique fissure
2. Inferior lobe
3. Superior lobe

Major Structures Related to the left lung

1. Rib I
2. Esophagus
3. Thoracic aorta
4. Diaphragm
5. Heart
6. Aortic arch
7. Left brachiocephalic vein
8. Left subclavian artery

1 _____
2 _____
3 _____
4 _____
5 _____

Major Structures Related to the Reft lung

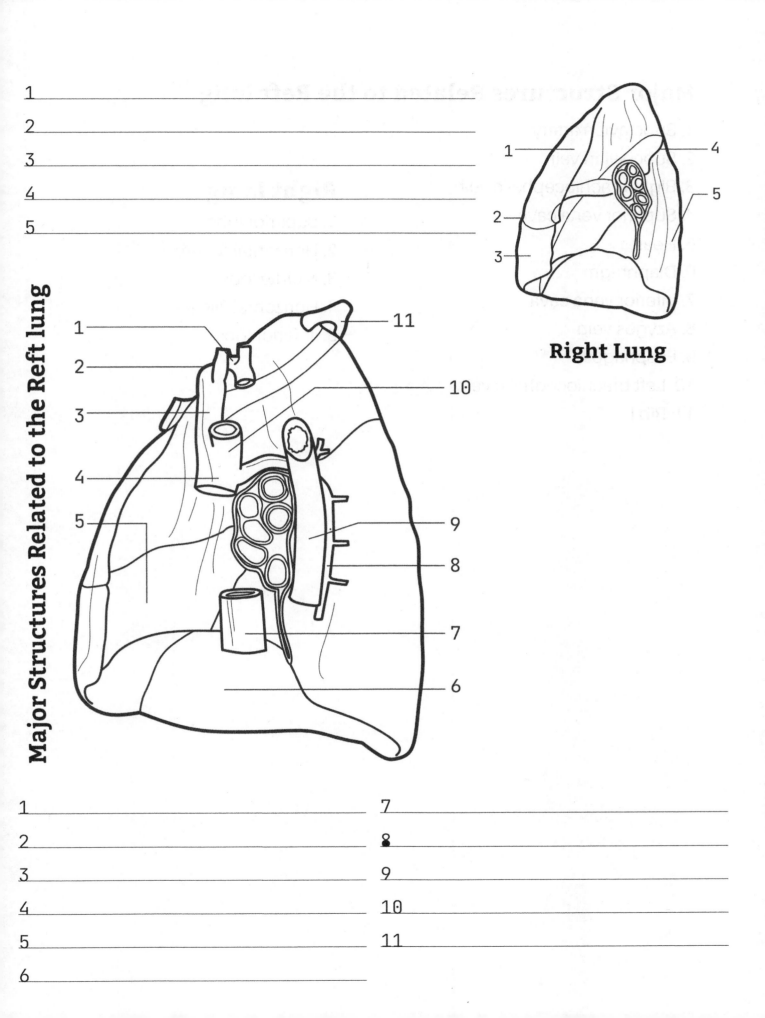

Right Lung

1 _____   7 _____
2 _____   8 _____
3 _____   9 _____
4 _____   10 _____
5 _____   11 _____
6 _____

Major Structures Related to the Reft lung

1. Subclavian artery
2. Subclavian vein
3. Right brachiocephalic vein
4. Superior vena cava
5. Heart
6. Diaphragm
7. Inferior vena cava
8. Azygos vein
9. Esophagus
10. Left brachiocephalic vein
11. Rib I

Right Lung

1. Superior lobe
2. Horizontal fissure
3. Middle lobe
4. Horizontal fissure
5. Inferior lobe

Wrist and Bones of the Hand

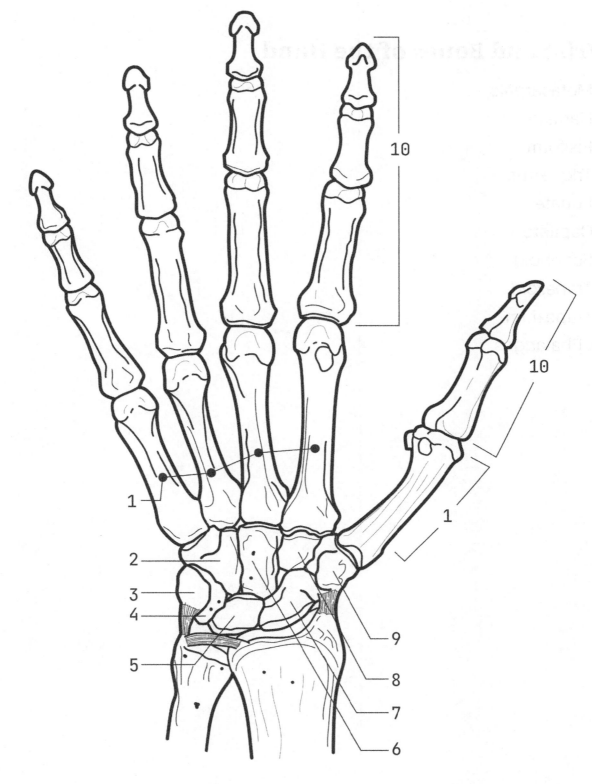

1 _____   6 _____

2 _____   7 _____

3 _____   8 _____

4 _____   9 _____

5 _____   10 _____

Wrist and Bones of the Hand

1. Metacarpals
2. Hamate
3. Pisiform
4. Triquetrum
5. Lunate
6. Capitate
7. Scaphoid
8. Trapezoid
9. Trapezium
10. Phalanges

Shoulder Joint

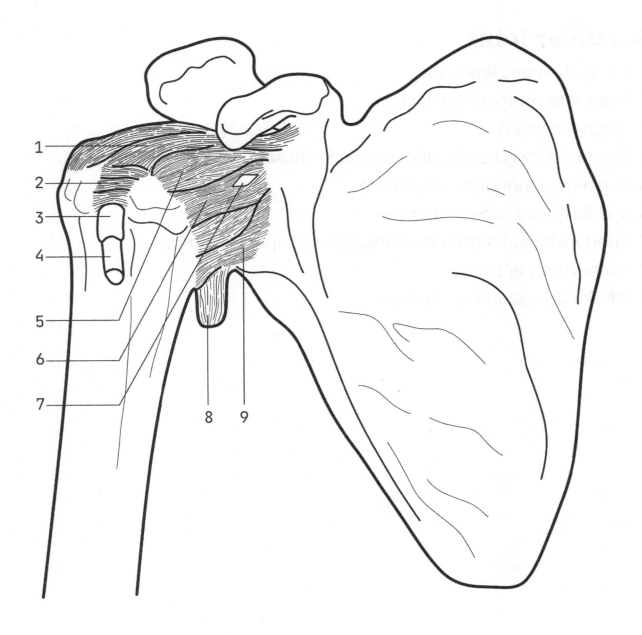

1 _____

2 _____

3 _____

4 _____

5 _____

6 _____

7 _____

8 _____

9 _____

Shoulder Joint

1. Coracohumeral ligament
2. Transverse humeral ligament
3. Synovial sheath
4. Tendon of long head of biceps brachii muscle
5. Superior glenohumeral ligament
6. Middle glenohumeral ligament
7. Aperture for subtendinous bursa of subscapularis muscle
8. Redundant capsule
9. Inferior glenohumeral ligament

Posterior View of Right Scapula

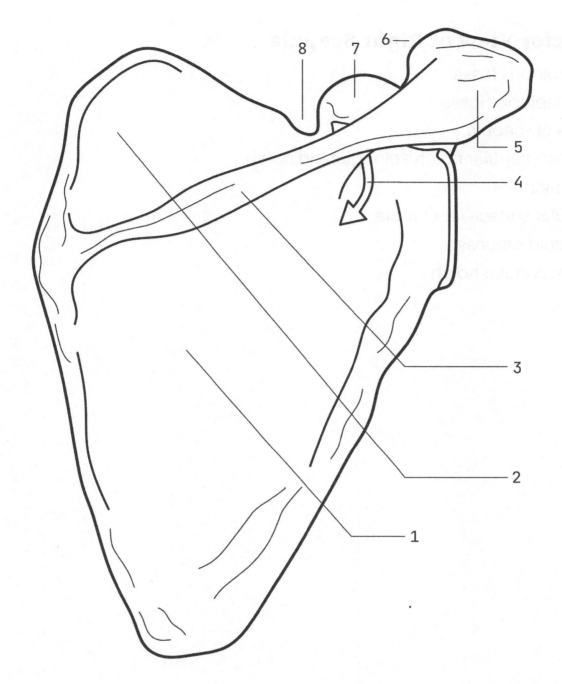

1 _____

2 _____

3 _____

4 _____

5 _____

6 _____

7 _____

8 _____

Posterior View of Right Scapula

1. Infraspinous fossa
2. Supraspinous fossa
3. Spine of scapula
4. Greater scapular notch/spinoglenoid notch
5. Acromion
6. Articular surface for clavicle
7. Coracoid process
8. Suprascapular notch

Scapula - Anterior view of costal surface

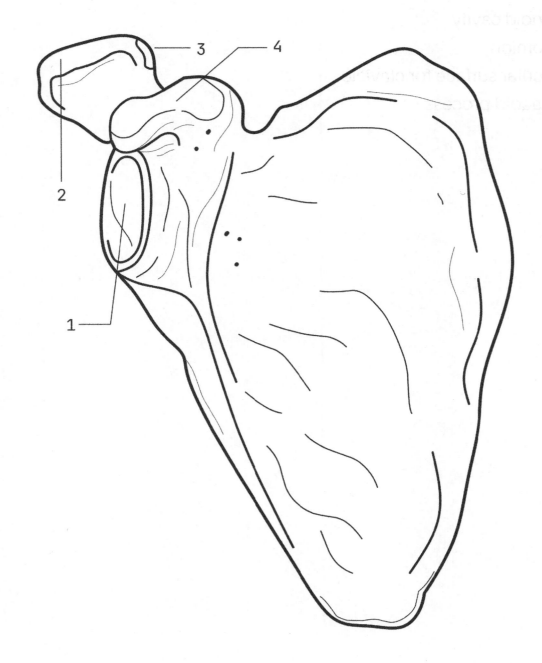

1 _____

2 _____

3 _____

4 _____

Scapula - Anterior View of Costal Surface

1. Glenoid cavity
2. Acromion
3. Articular surface for clavicle
4. Coracoid process

Bones of the Upper Limb

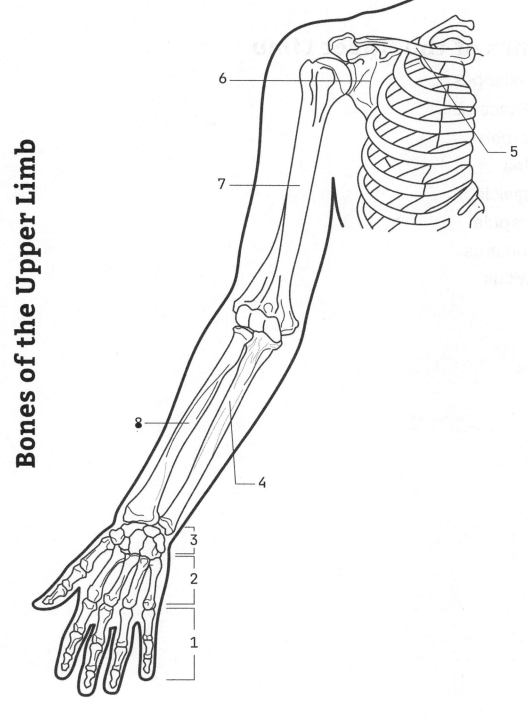

1 _____

2 _____

3 _____

4 _____

5 _____

6 _____

7 _____

8 _____

Bones of the Upper Limb

1. Phalanges
2. Metacarpals
3. Carpals
4. Ulna
5. Clavicle
6. Scapula
7. Humerus
8. Radius

Elbow Joint

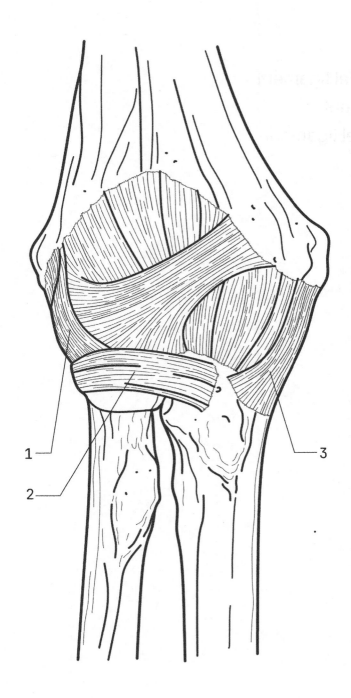

1 _____

2 _____

3 _____

1 _____

2 _____

3 _____

Elbow Joint

1. Radial collateral ligament
2. Annular ligament
3. Ulnar collateral ligament

Humerus (Posterior View)

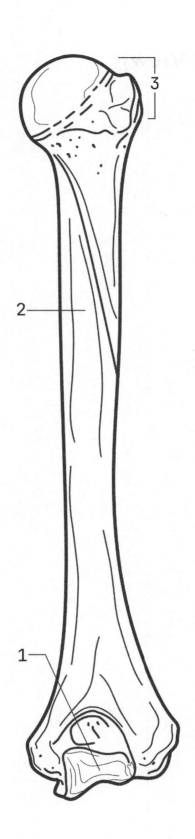

1 _____

2 _____

3 _____

Humerus (Posterior View)

1. Trochlea
2. Radial groove
3. Greater tubercle

Proximal End of Right Humerus

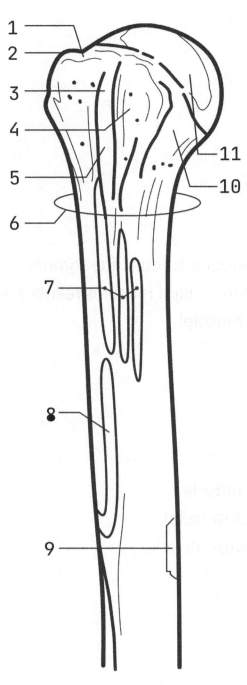

Anterior View

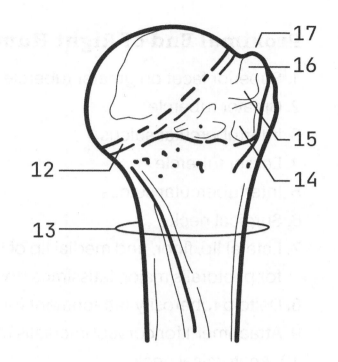

Posterior View

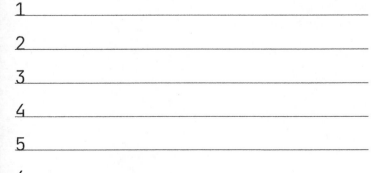

1 _____

2 _____

3 _____

4 _____

5 _____

6 _____

7 _____

8 _____

9 _____

10 _____

11 _____

12 _____

13 _____

14 _____

15 _____

16 _____

17 _____

Proximal End of Right Humerus

1. Superior facet on greater tubercle

2. Greater tubercle

3. Intertubercular sulcus

4. Lesser tubercle

5. Intertubercular sulcus

6. Surgical neck

7. Lateral lip, floor, and medial lip of intertubercular sulcus (attachment for pectoralis major, latissimus dorsi, and teres major muscles respectively).

8. Deltoid tuberosity (attachment for deltoid muscle)

9. Attachment for coracobrachialis muscle

10. Anatomical neck

11. Head

12. Anatomical neck

13. Surgical neck

14. Inferior facet (attachment for teres minor muscle)

15. Middle facet (attachment for infraspinatus muscle)

16. Superior facet (attachment for supraspinatus muscle)

17. Greater tubercle

Proximal End of Ulna

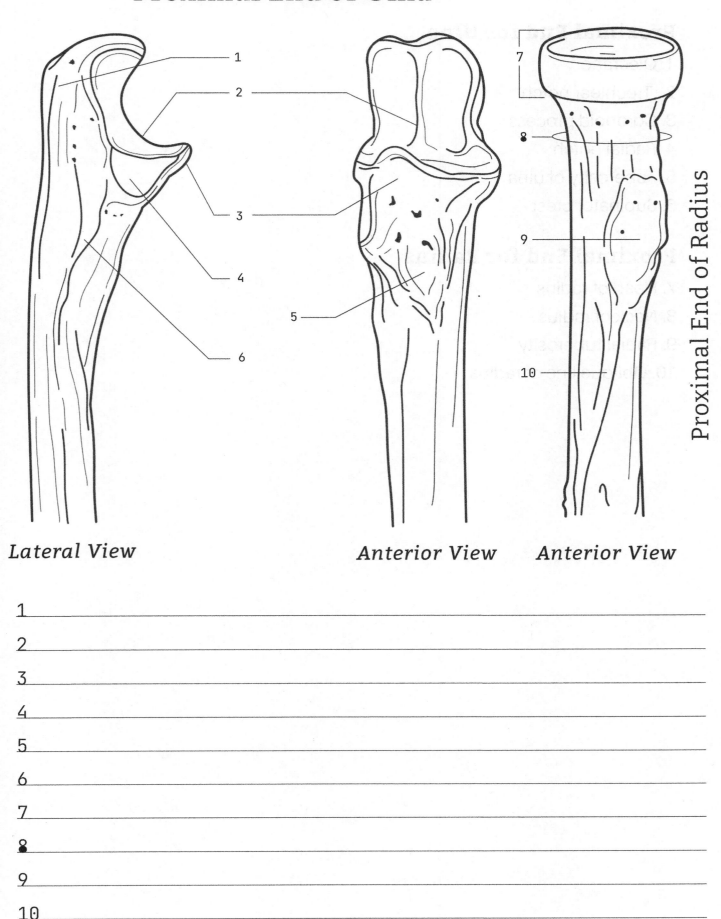

Lateral View

Anterior View

Anterior View

Proximal End of Radius

1 _____

2 _____

3 _____

4 _____

5 _____

6 _____

7 _____

8 _____

9 _____

10 _____

Proximal End for Ulna

1. Olecranon
2. Trochlear notch
3. Coronoid process
4. Radial notch
5. Tuberosity of ulna
6. Supinator crest

Proximal End for Radius

7. Head of radius
8. Neck of radius
9. Radial tuberosity
10. Oblique line of radius

Layers of the Abdominal Wall

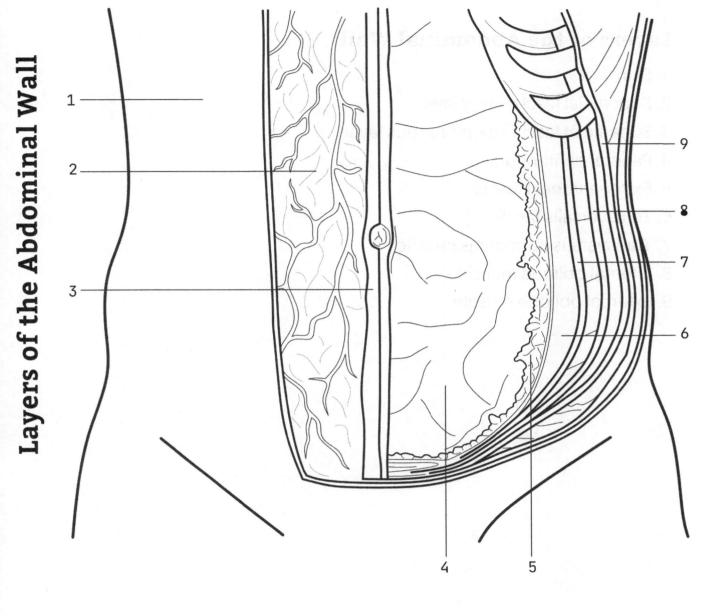

1 _____

2 _____

3 _____

4 _____

5 _____

6 _____

7 _____

8 _____

9 _____

Layers of the Abdominal Wall

1. Skin
2. Superficial fascia - fatty layer
3. Superficial fascia - membranous layer
4. Parietal peritoneum
5. Extraperitoneal fascia
6. Transversalis fascia
7. Transversus abdominis muscle
8. Internal oblique muscle
9. External oblique muscle

Large Intestine

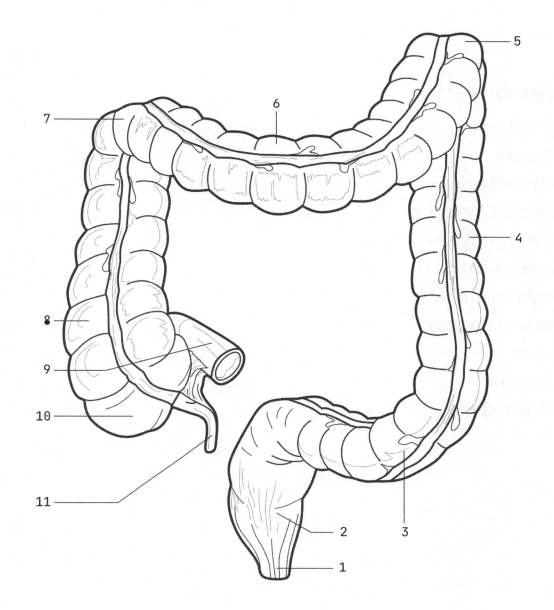

1 _____

2 _____

3 _____

4 _____

5 _____

6 _____

7 _____

8 _____

9 _____

10 _____

11 _____

Large Intestine

1. Anal canal
2. Rectum
3. Sigmoid colon
4. Descending colon
5. Left colic flexure
6. Transverse colon
7. Right colic flexure
8. Ascending colon
9. Ileum
10. Cecum
11. Appendix

Rectus Abdominis

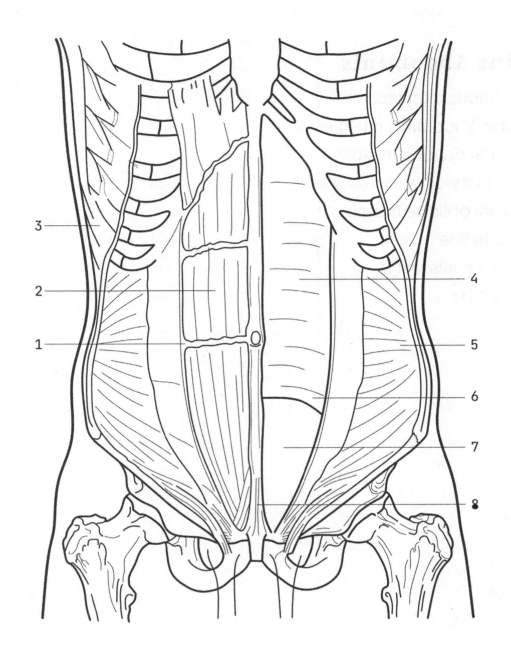

1 _____

2 _____

3 _____

4 _____

5 _____

6 _____

7 _____

8 _____

Rectus Abdominis

1. Tendinous intersection
2. Rectus abdominis muscle
3. External oblique muscle
4. Posterior wall of rectus sheath
5. Internal oblique muscle
6. Arcuate line
7. Transversalis fascia
8. Linea alba

Duodenum

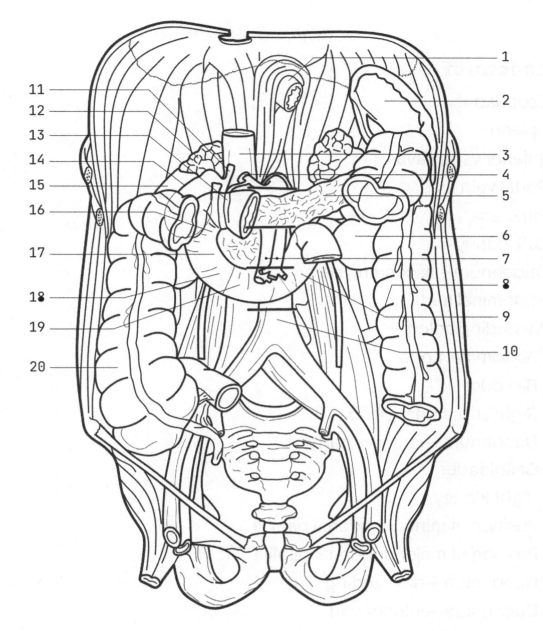

1 _____   11 _____

2 _____   12 _____

3 _____   13 _____

4 _____   14 _____

5 _____   15 _____

6 _____   16 _____

7 _____   17 _____

8 _____   18 _____

9 _____   19 _____

10 _____   20 _____

Duodenum

1. Esophagus
2. Spleen
3. Inferior vena cava
4. Portal vein
5. Pancreas
6. Left kidney
7. Duodenum—ascending part
8. Abdominal aorta
9. Ascending colon
10. Abdominal aorta
11. Bile duct
12. Right suprarenal gland
13. Duodenum—superior part
14. Gallbladder
15. Right kidney
16. Position of minor duodenal papilla
17. Position of major duodenal papilla
18. Duodenum—descending part
19. Duodenum—inferior part
20. Ascending colon

Internal Structure Of the Kidney

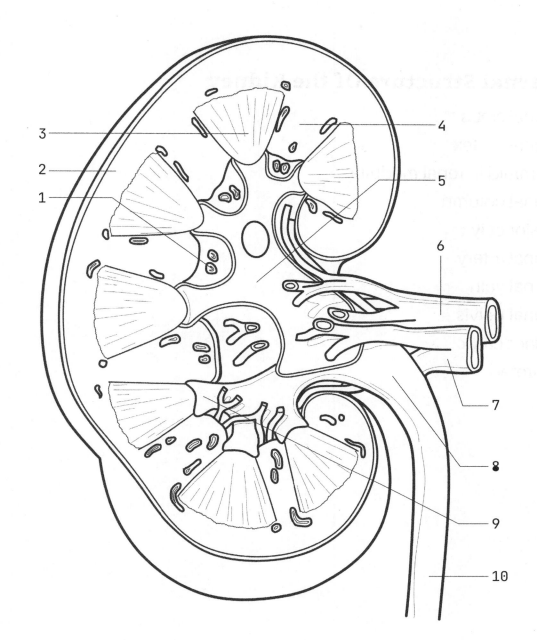

1 _____

2 _____

3 _____

4 _____

5 _____

6 _____

7 _____

8 _____

9 _____

10 _____

Internal Structure Of the Kidney

1. Renal sinus
2. Renal cortex
3. Pyramid in renal medulla
4. Renal column
5. Major calyx
6. Renal artery
7. Renal vein
8. Renal pelvis
9. Minor calyx
10. Ureter

Abdominal Wall - Transverse Section

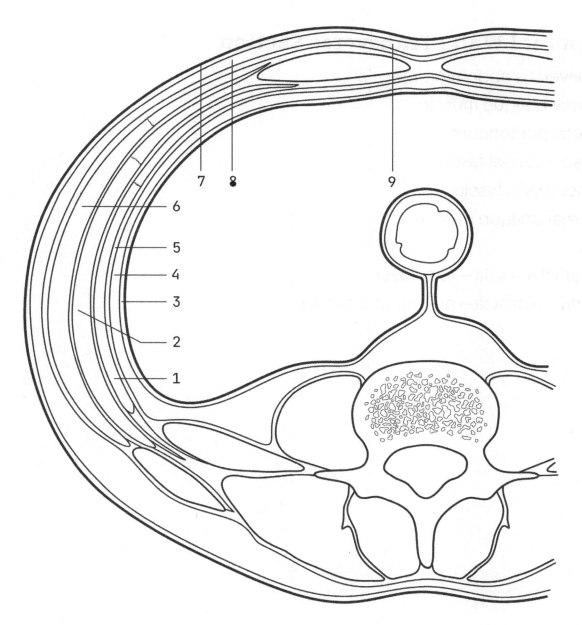

1 _____

2 _____

3 _____

4 _____

5 _____

6 _____

7 _____

8 _____

9 _____

Abdominal Wall - Transverse Section

1. Transversus abdominis muscle
2. Internal oblique muscle
3. Parietal peritoneum
4. Extraperitoneal fascia
5. Transversalis fascia
6. External oblique muscle
7. Skin
8. Superficial fascia—fatty layer
9. Superficial fascia—membranous layer

Bile Drainage

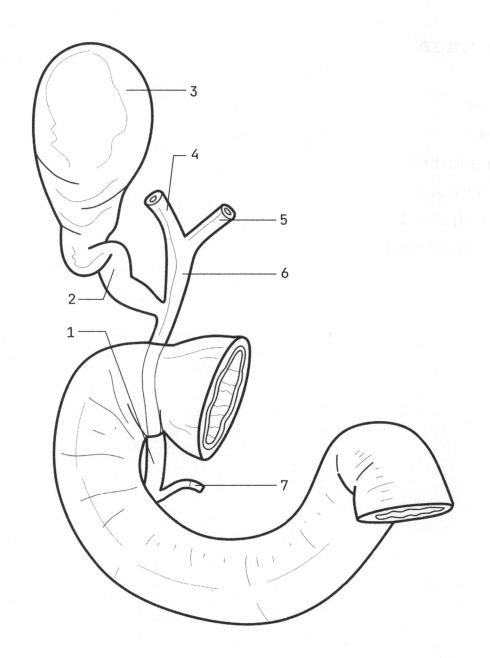

1 _____

2 _____

3 _____

4 _____

5 _____

6 _____

7 _____

Bile Drainage

1. Bile duct
2. Cystic duct
3. Gallbladder
4. Right hepatic duct
5. Left hepatic duct
6. Common hepatic duct
7. Main pancreatic duct

Osteology of the Posterior Abdominal wall

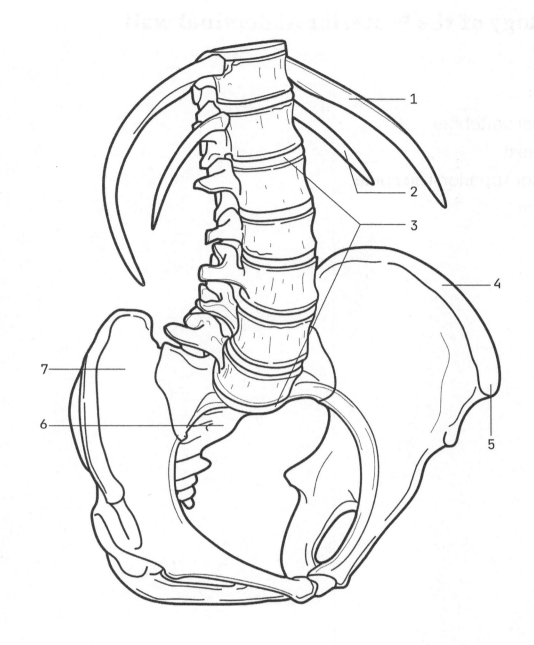

1 _____

2 _____

3 _____

4 _____

5 _____

6 _____

7 _____

Osteology of the Posterior Abdominal wall

1. Rib XI
2. Rib XII
3. Lumbar vertebrae
4. Iliac crest
5. Anterior superior iliac spine
6. Sacrum
7. Ilium

Spermatic Cord

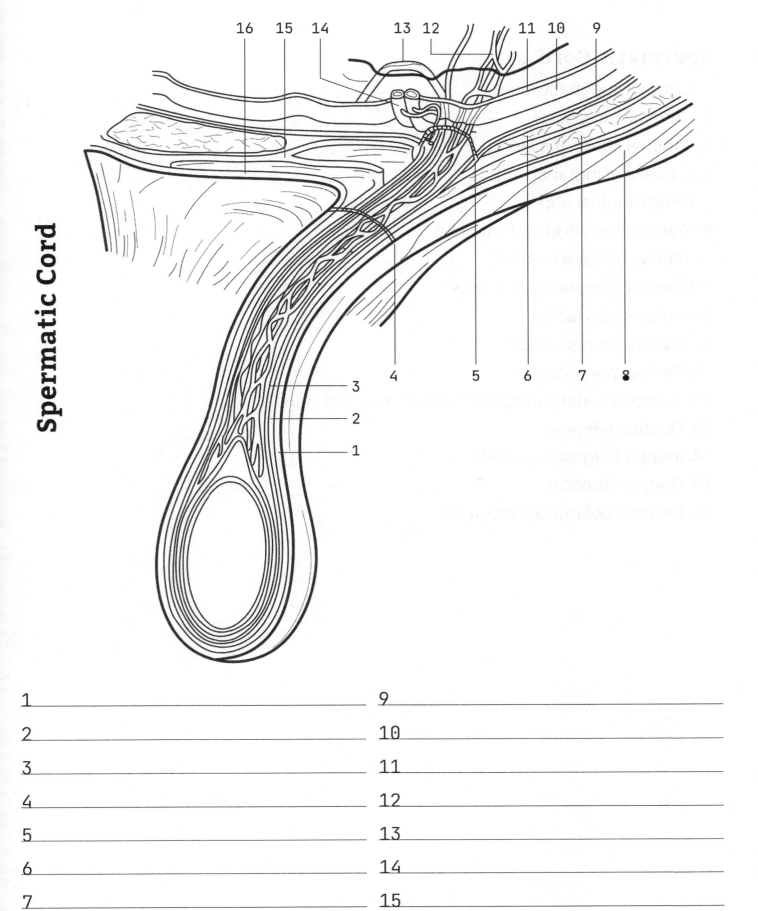

1 _____

2 _____

3 _____

4 _____

5 _____

6 _____

7 _____

8 _____

9 _____

10 _____

11 _____

12 _____

13 _____

14 _____

15 _____

16 _____

Spermatic Cord

1. External spermatic fascia
2. Cremasteric fascia
3. Internal spermatic fascia
4. Superficial inguinal ring
5. Deep inguinal ring
6. Transversus abdominis muscle
7. Internal oblique muscle
8. External oblique aponeurosis
9. Transversalis fascia
10. Extraperitoneal fascia
11. Parietal peritoneum
12. Testicular artery and pampiniform plexus of veins
13. Ductus deferens
14. Inferior epigastric vessels
15. Conjoint tendon
16. External oblique aponeurosis

The Stomach

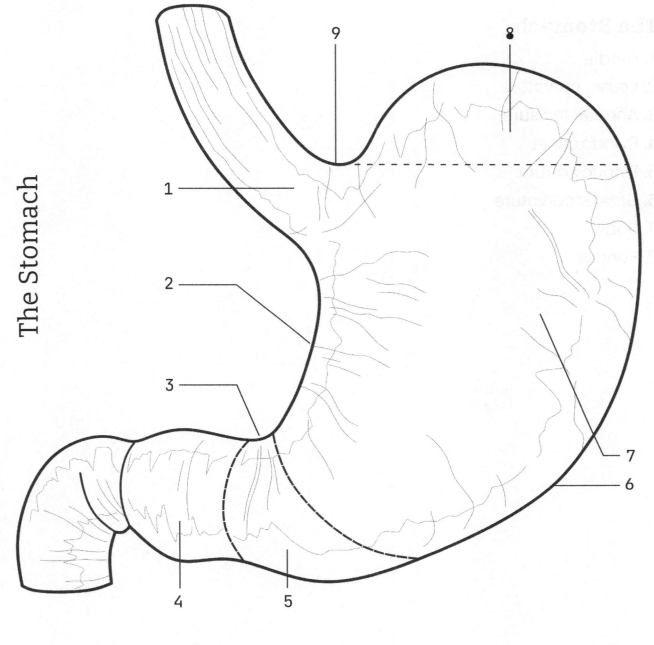

1 _____

2 _____

3 _____

4 _____

5 _____

6 _____

7 _____

8 _____

9 _____

The Stomach

1. Cardia
2. Lesser curvature
3. Angular incisure
4. Pyloric canal
5. Pyloric antrum
6. Greater curvature
7. Body
8. Fundus

The Lever

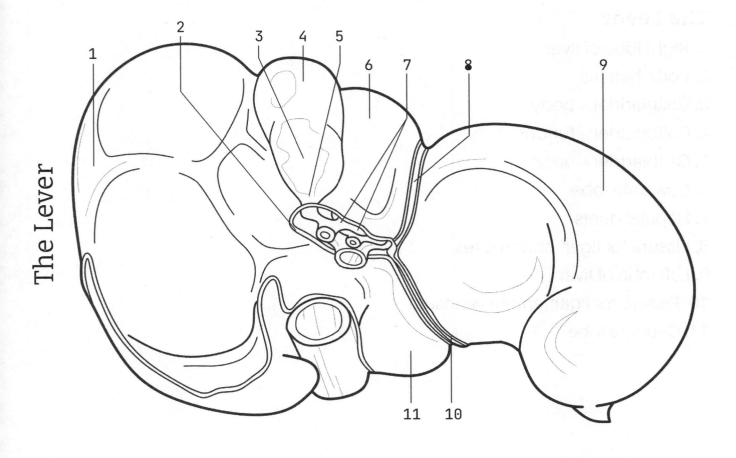

1 _____

2 _____

3 _____

4 _____

5 _____

6 _____

7 _____

8 _____

9 _____

10 _____

11 _____

The Lever

1. Right lobe of liver
2. Porta hepatis
3. Gallbladder – body
4. Gallbladder – fundus
5. Gallbladder – neck
6. Quadrate lobe
7. Hepatic ducts
8. Fissure for ligamentum teres
9. Left lobe of liver
10. Fissure for ligamentum venosum
11. Caudate lobe

Bones of the Foot - Dorsal View

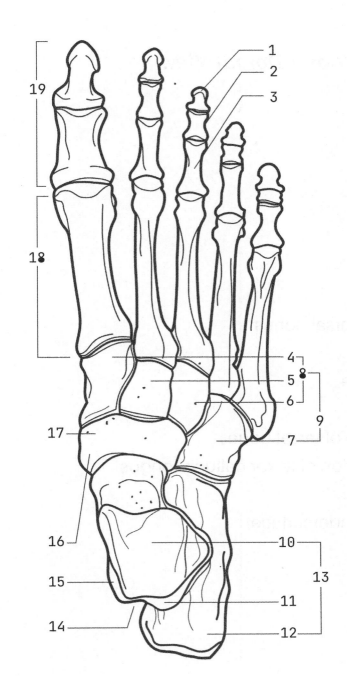

1 _____   11 _____

2 _____   12 _____

3 _____   13 _____

4 _____   14 _____

5 _____   15 _____

6 _____   16 _____

7 _____   17 _____

8 _____   18 _____

9 _____   19 _____

10 _____

Bones of the Foot - *Dorsal View*

1. Distal
2. Middle
3. Proximal
4. Medial
5. Intermediate
6. Lateral
7. Cuboid
8. Cuneiforms
9. Distal group of tarsal bones
10. Talus
11. Lateral tubercle
12. Calcaneus
13. Proximal group of tarsal bones
14. Groove for tendon of flexor hallucis longus
15. Medial tubercle
16. Tubercle (on undersurface)
17. Navicular
18. Metatarsals
19. Phalanges

Ligaments of the Ankle Joint

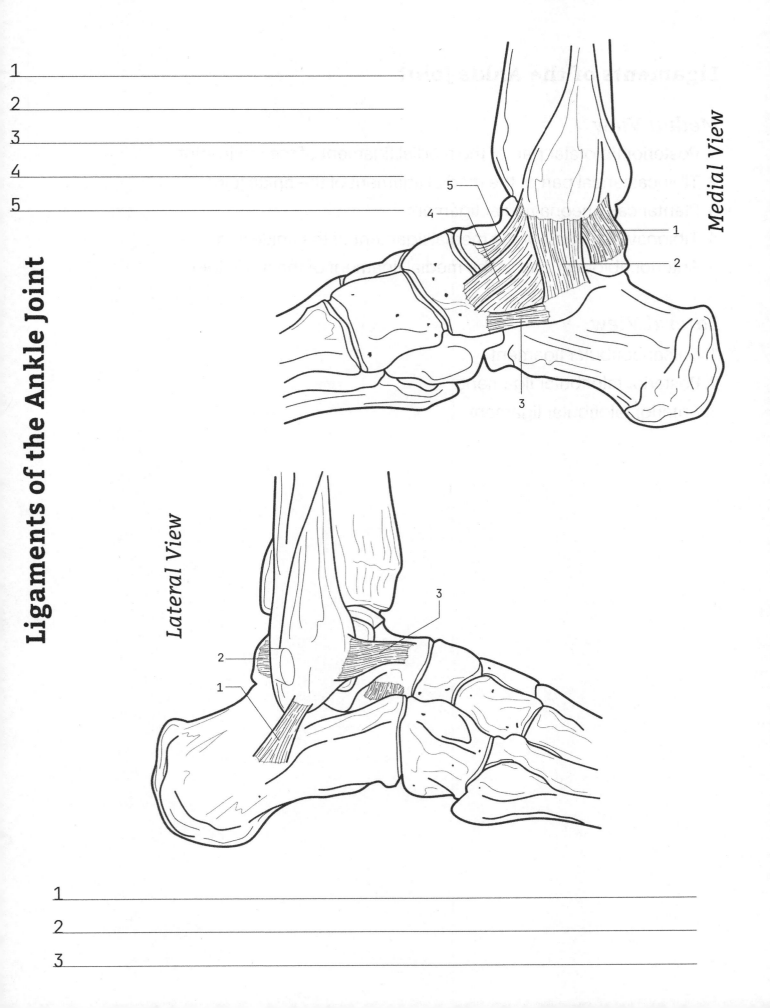

1 _____

2 _____

3 _____

4 _____

5 _____

Medial View

Lateral View

1 _____

2 _____

3 _____

Ligaments of the Ankle Joint

Medial View

1. Posterior tibiotalar part of the medial ligament of the ankle joint
2. Tibiocalcaneal part of the medial ligament of the ankle joint
3. Plantar calcaneonavicular ligament
4. Tibionavicular part of the medial ligament of the ankle joint
5. Anterior tibiotalar part of the medial ligament of the ankle joint

Lateral View

1. Calcaneofibular ligament
2. Posterior talofibular ligament
3. Anterior talofibular ligament

Ischiofemoral Ligament (*Posterior View*)

1 _____

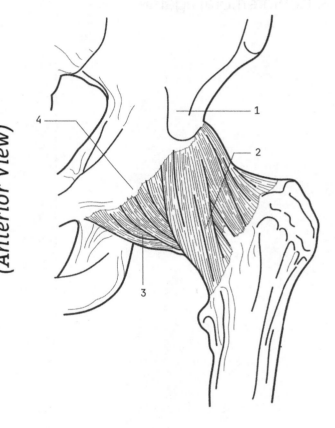

Iliofemoral and Pubofemoral Ligaments (*Anterior View*)

1 _____

2 _____

3 _____

Iliofemoral and Pubofemoral Ligaments
(Anterior View)

1. Anterior inferior iliac spine
2. Iliofemoral ligament
3. Pubofemoral ligament
4. Iliopubic eminence

Ischiofemoral Ligament *(Posterior View)*

1. Ischiofemoral ligament

Bones and Joints of the Lower Limb

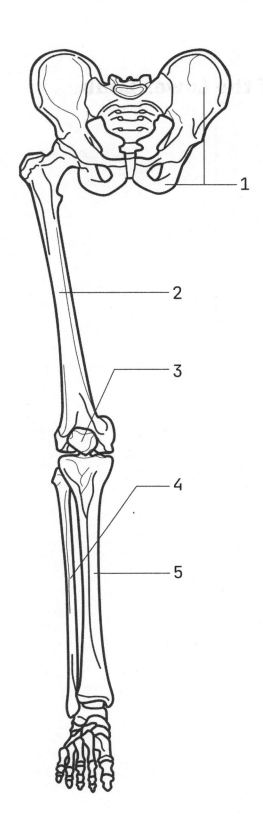

1 _____

2 _____

3 _____

4 _____

5 _____

Bones and Joints of the Lower Limb

1. Pelvic bone
2. Femur
3. Patella
4. Fibula
5. Tibia

Acetabulum

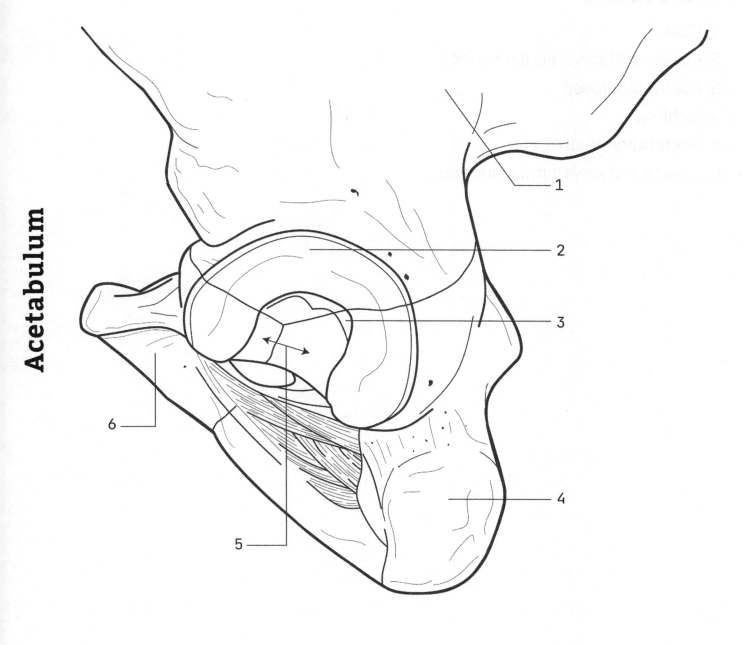

1 _____

2 _____

3 _____

4 _____

5 _____

6 _____

Acetabulum

1. Ilium
2. Lunate surface/articular surface
3. Acetabular fossa
4. Ischium
5. Acetabular notch
6. Lunate surface/articular surface

Tibia and Fibula

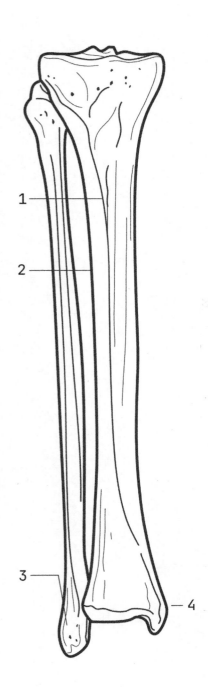

Anterior View

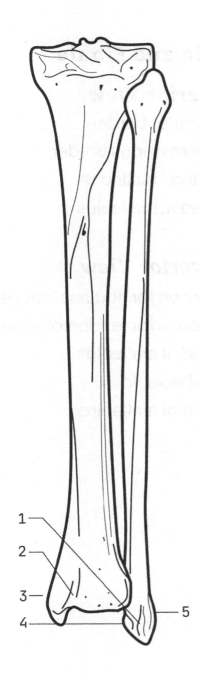

Posterior View

1 _____

2 _____

3 _____

4 _____

1 _____

2 _____

3 _____

4 _____

5 _____

Tibia and Fibula

Anterior View

1. Anterior border
2. Interosseous border
3. Lateral malleolus
4. Medial malleolus

Posterior View

1. Groove for fibularis longus and brevis muscles
2. Groove for tendon of tibialis posterior muscle
3. Medial malleolus
4. Malleolar fossa
5. Lateral malleolus

Proximal End of the Femur

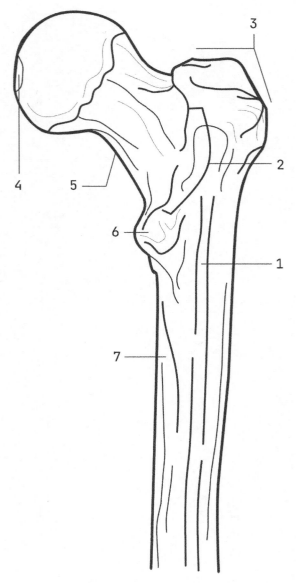

Posterior View

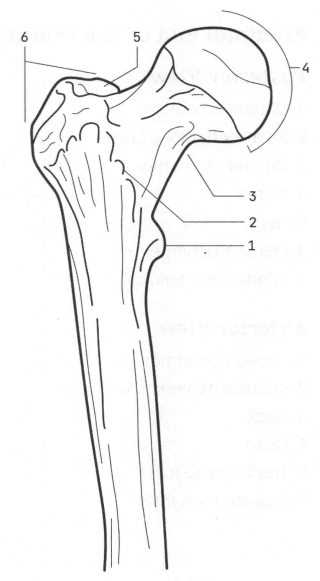

Anterior View

1 _____

2 _____

3 _____

4 _____

5 _____

6 _____

7 _____

1 _____

2 _____

3 _____

4 _____

5 _____

6 _____

Proximal End of the Femur

Posterior View

1. Gluteal tuberosity
2. Intertrochanteric crest
3. Greater trochanter
4. Fovea
5. Neck
6. Lesser trochanter
7. Intertrochanteric crest

Anterior View

1. Lesser trochanter
2. Intertrochanteric line
3. Neck
4. Head
5. Trochanteric fossa
6. Greater trochanter

Knee Joint
(Joint capsule is not shown)

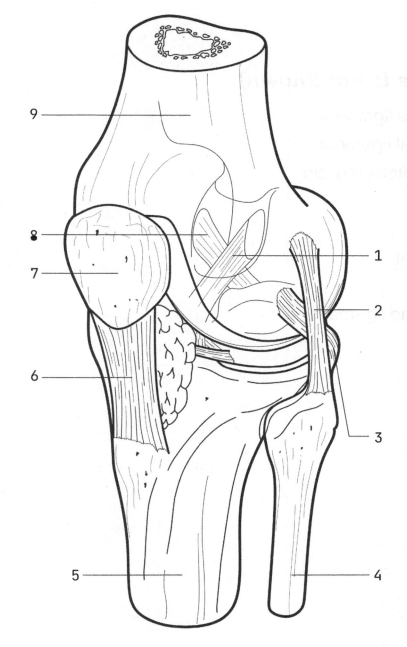

1 _____

2 _____

3 _____

4 _____

5 _____

6 _____

7 _____

8 _____

9 _____

Knee Joint
(Joint Capsule is not Shown)

1. Anterior cruciate ligament
2. Fibular collateral ligament
3. Tendon of popliteus muscle
4. Fibula
5. Tibia
6. Patellar ligament
7. Patella
8. Posterior cruciate ligament
9. Femur

Collateral Ligaments of the Knee Joint

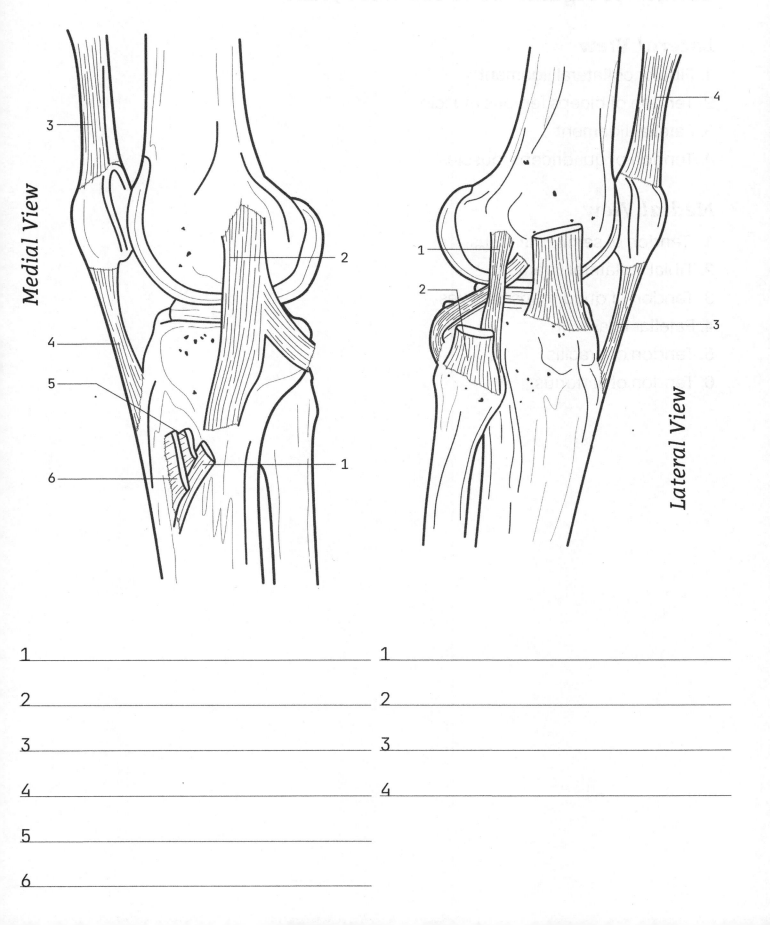

Medial View

Lateral View

1 _____   1 _____

2 _____   2 _____

3 _____   3 _____

4 _____   4 _____

5 _____

6 _____

Collateral Ligaments of the Knee Joint

Lateral View

1. Fibular collateral ligament
2. Tendon of biceps femoris muscle
3. Patellar ligament
4. Tendon of quadriceps muscles

Medial View

1. Tendon of semitendinosus
2. Tibial collateral ligament
3. Tendon of quadriceps muscles
4. Patellar ligament
5. Tendon of gracilis
6. Tendon of sartorius

Articular Surface of the Knee Joint

1 _____

2 _____

3 _____

4 _____

Anterior View

Menisci of the Knee Joint

Superior View

1 _____

2 _____

3 _____

4 _____

5 _____

6 _____

7 _____

8 _____

Articular Surface of the Knee Joint

Anterior View

1. Patella
2. Surface for articulation with patella
3. Flat surfaces for articulation with tibia in extension
4. Intercondylar region
5. Posterior cruciate ligament
6. Round surfaces for articulation with tibia in flexion
7. Meniscus
8. Anterior cruciate ligament

Menisci of the Knee Joint
Superior View

1. Posterior cruciate ligament
2. Medial meniscus
3. Flat surfaces for articulation with tibia in extension
4. Lateral meniscus

Female Perineum

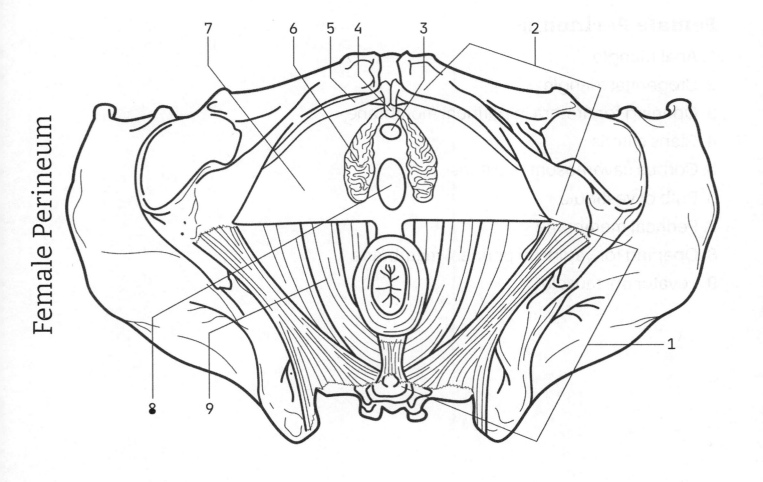

1 _____

2 _____

3 _____

4 _____

5 _____

6 _____

7 _____

8 _____

9 _____

Female Perineum

1. Anal triangle
2. Urogenital triangle
3. Opening for urethra in perineal membrane
4. Glans clitoris
5. Corpus cavernosum of clitoris
6. Bulb of vestibule
7. Perineal membrane
8. Opening for vagina in perineal membrane
9. Levator ani muscle

Male Perineum

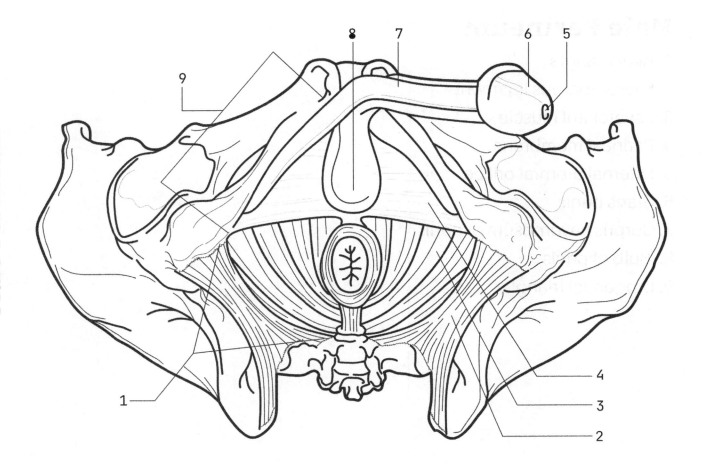

1 _____

2 _____

3 _____

4 _____

5 _____

6 _____

7 _____

8 _____

9 _____

Male Perineum

1. Anal triangle
2. Sacrotuberous ligament
3. Levator ani muscle
4. Perineal membrane
5. External urethral orifice
6. Glans penis
7. Corpus cavernosum of penis
8. Bulb of penis
9. Urogenital triangle

Female Reproductive System

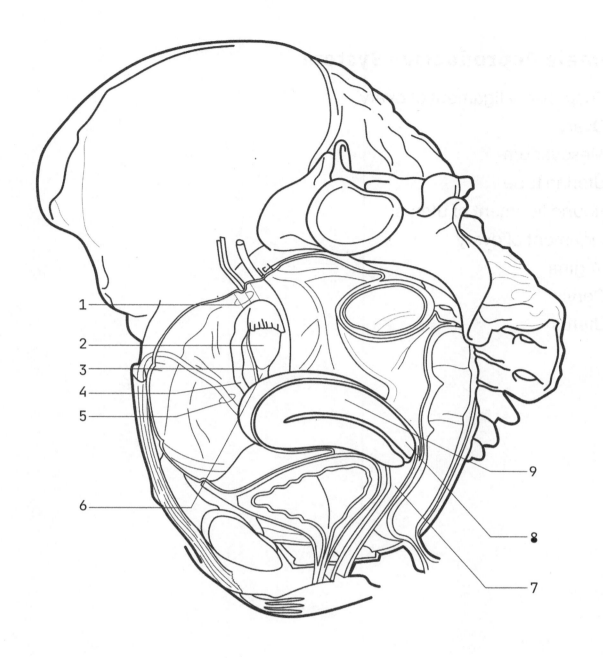

1 _____

2 _____

3 _____

4 _____

5 _____

6 _____

7 _____

8 _____

9 _____

Female Reproductive System

1. Suspensory ligament of ovary
2. Ovary
3. Mesovarium
4. Uterine tube
5. Round ligament of uterus
6. Ligament of ovary
7. Vagina
8. Cervix
9. Uterus

Male Reproductive System

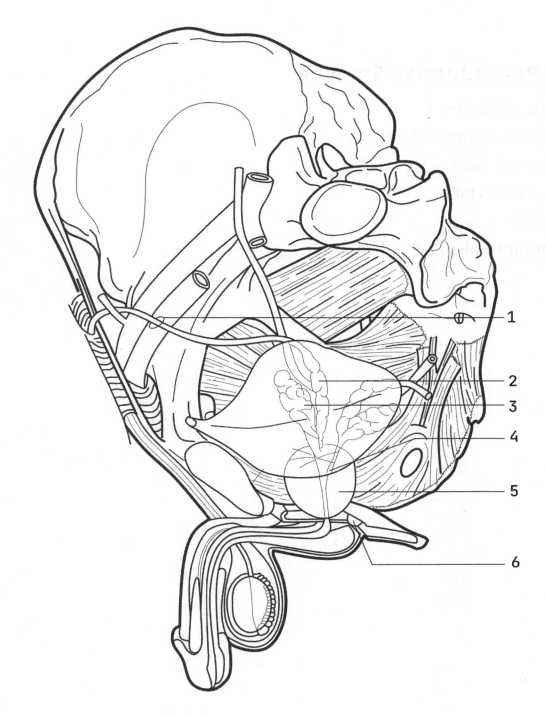

1 _____

2 _____

3 _____

4 _____

5 _____

6 _____

Male Reproductive System

1. Ductus deferens
2. Ampulla of ductus deferens
3. Seminal vesicle
4. Ejaculatory duct
5. Prostate
6. Bulbourethral gland

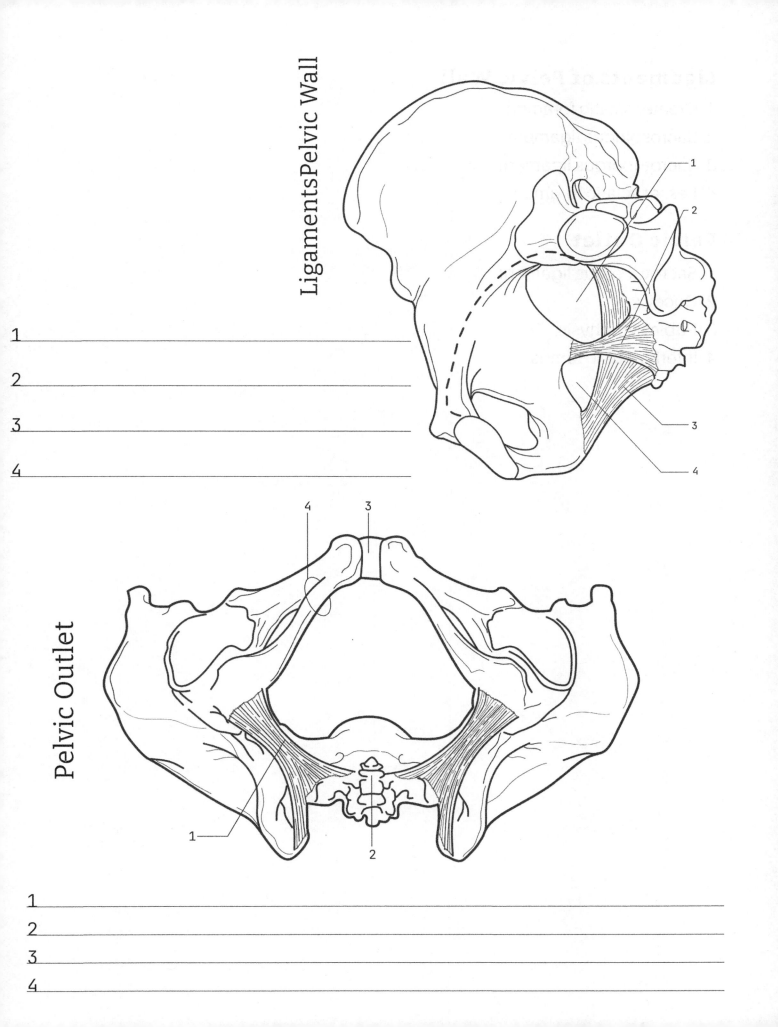

1 _____

2 _____

3 _____

4 _____

Pelvic Outlet

1 _____

2 _____

3 _____

4 _____

Ligaments of Pelvic Wall

1. Greater sciatic foramen
2. Sacrospinous ligament
3. Sacrotuberous ligament
4. Lesser sciatic foramen

Pelvic Outlet

1. Sacrotuberous ligament
2. Coccyx
3. Pubic symphysis
4. Inferior pubic ramus

Pelvic Bone

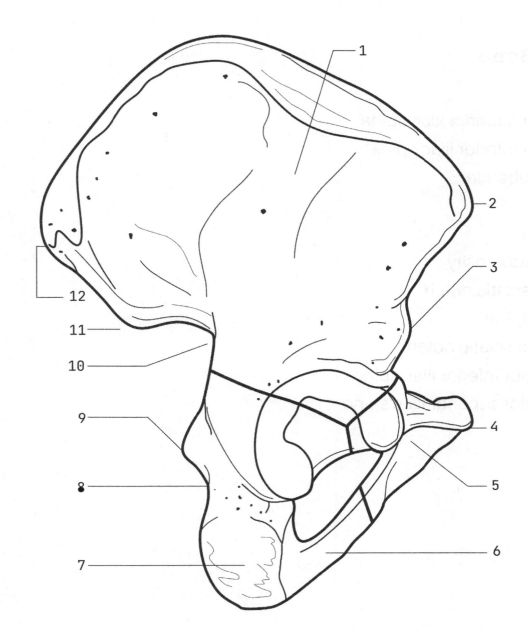

1 _____
2 _____
3 _____
4 _____
5 _____
6 _____
7 _____
8 _____
9 _____
10 _____
11 _____
12 _____

Pelvic Bone

1. Ilium
2. Anterior superior iliac spine
3. Anterior inferior iliac spine
4. Pubic tubercle
5. Pubis
6. Ischium
7. Ischial tuberosity
8. Lesser sciatic notch
9. Ischial spine
10. Greater sciatic notch
11. Posterior inferior iliac spine
12. Posterior superior iliac spine

Pelvis

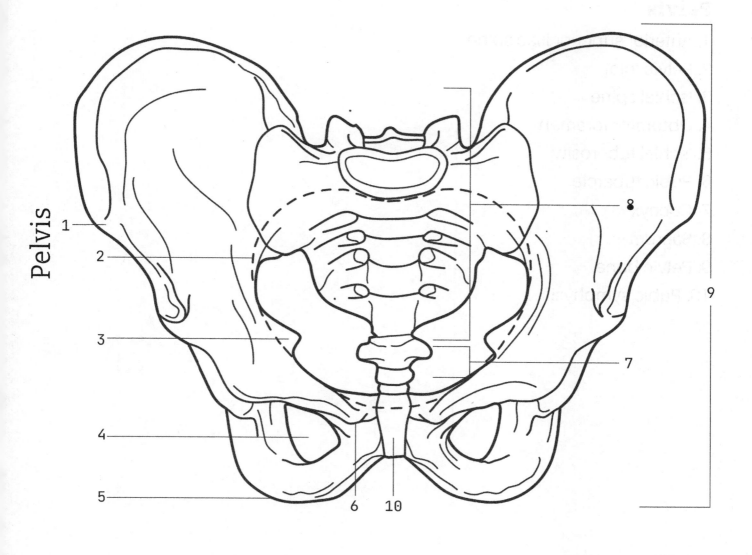

1 _____

2 _____

3 _____

4 _____

5 _____

6 _____

7 _____

8 _____

9 _____

10 _____

Pelvis

1. Anterior superior iliac spine
2. Pelvic inlet
3. Ischial spine
4. Obturator foramen
5. Ischial tuberosity
6. Pubic tubercle
7. Coccyx
8. Sacrum
9. Pelvic bone
10. Pubic symphysis

Uterine Tube

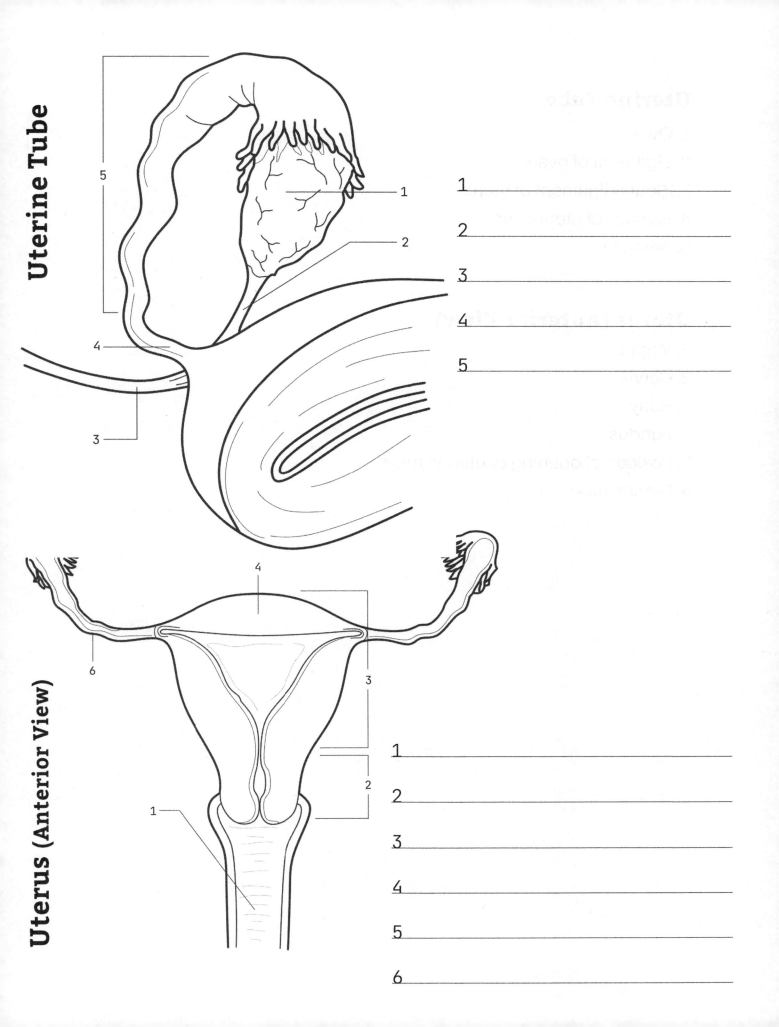

1 _____

2 _____

3 _____

4 _____

5 _____

Uterus (Anterior View)

1 _____

2 _____

3 _____

4 _____

5 _____

6 _____

Uterine Tube

1. Ovary
2. Ligament of ovary
3. Round ligament of uterus
4. Isthmus of uterine tube
5. Ampulla

Uterus (Anterior View)

1. Vagina
2. Cervix
3. Body
4. Fundus
5. Position of opening of uterine tube
6. Uterine tube

Viscera - Female Overview

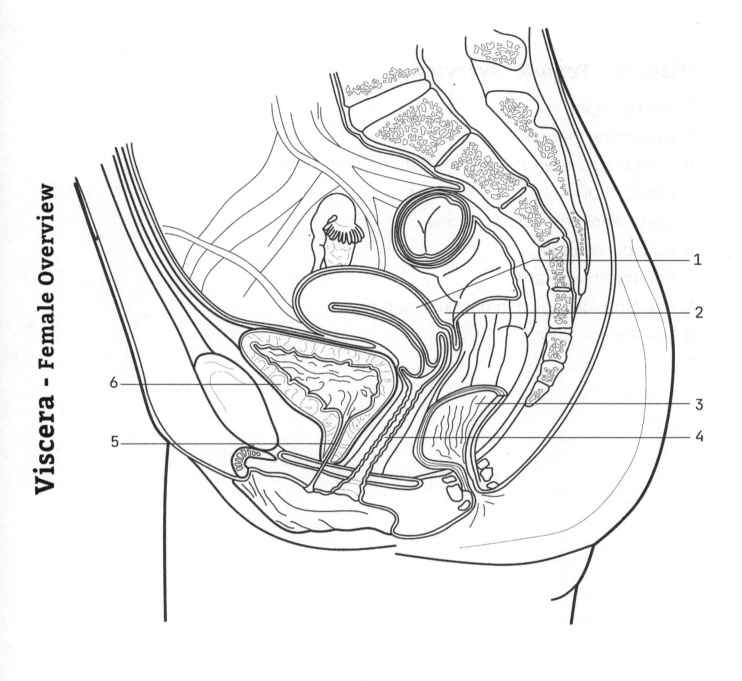

1 _____

2 _____

3 _____

4 _____

5 _____

6 _____

Viscera - *Female Overview*

1. Anal triangle
2. Urogenital triangle
3. Opening for urethra in perineal membrane
4. Glans clitoris
5. Corpus cavernosum of clitoris
6. Bulb of vestibule
7. Perineal membrane
8. Opening for vagina in perineal membrane
9. Levator ani muscle

Viscera - Male Overview

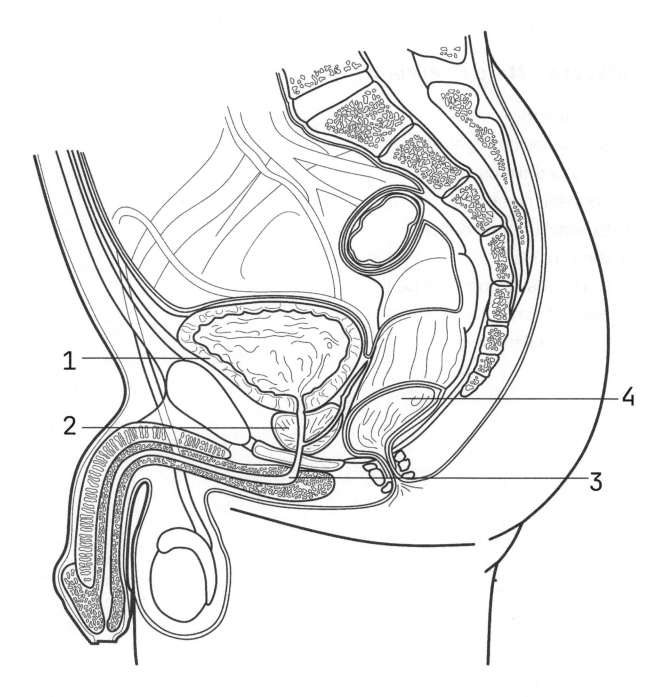

1
2
3
4

1 _____

2 _____

3 _____

4 _____

Viscera - *Male Overview*

1. Anal triangle
2. Sacrotuberous ligament
3. Levator ani muscle
4. Perineal membrane
5. External urethral orifice
6. Glans penis
7. Corpus cavernosum of penis
8. Bulb of penis
9. Urogenital triangle

Made in United States
North Haven, CT
20 December 2024

63186174R00065